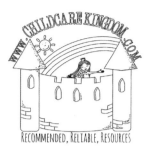

SAFER FOOD
BETTER BUSINESS

FOR CHILDMINDERS

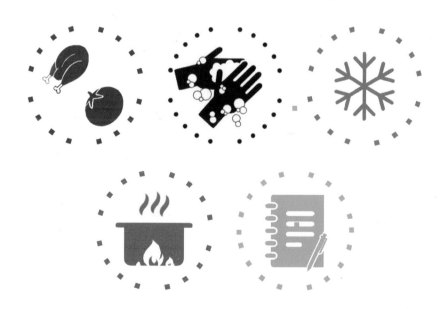

Updated: December 2015

HOW TO USE THIS PACK

Welcome to Safer food, better business for childminders

IS THIS PACK FOR ME?

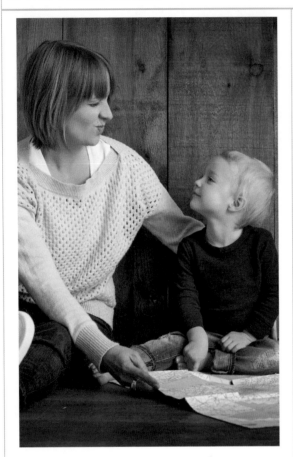

This pack is for you if you are a registered childminder or childcarer on domestic premises (where you look after children in your home) and you usually provide meals and drinks for the children in your care. It will help you comply with the law.

Do you usually:

- provide meals, snacks or drinks (apart from mains tap water) for children or babies?

  Yes ☐   No ☐

  and / or

- reheat food provided by a parent / carer, or cut it up?

  Yes ☐   No ☐

If you said **yes** to one or both of these questions, then this pack is for you. If you provide food for children in your care, you must comply with food safety and hygiene regulations.

If you think this pack does not cover all the food preparation and cooking you do, contact the environmental health department at your local authority for advice.

If **no** (you don't usually do either of these things) and you just do the following, you do not have to use this pack:

- keep packed lunches in your fridge that are brought by parents / carers

  and / or

- provide plates and cutlery for the children to use to eat their own packed lunches

  and / or

- only provide food occasionally, e.g. a birthday cake for one of the children, or if a parent/carer has been delayed in picking up a child

If you are not sure whether to use this pack, contact the environmental health department at your local authority for advice.

Home childcarers and nannies who look after children in the child's home do not need to use this pack.

If you run childcare on non-domestic premises, e.g. a nursery, you should use the pack called 'Safer food, better business for caterers'. However, you may find some of the information in this pack useful, e.g. the advice on feeding babies and children.

HOW DOES THIS PACK HELP ME COMPLY WITH THE LAW?

Food safety and hygiene regulations say that you must be able to show what you do to make sure the food you provide for children and babies is safe to eat. You must also have this written down and the pack helps you to do this.

This pack is based on the principles of HACCP (hazard analysis and critical control point), but you will not find words such as 'HACCP' or 'hazard' in the pack because we have cut out all the jargon.

The pack has been developed by the Food Standards Agency to be practical and easy to use, with as little paperwork as possible.

There are also food hygiene requirements in the Statutory Framework for the Early Years Foundation stage and other regulations that form part of your registration as a childminder / childcarer.

In England you can get further information on these from Ofsted (the Office for Standards in Education, Children's Services and Skills) or in Wales from the Care and Social Services Inspectorate Wales or in Scotland from the Care Inspectorate. These requirements do not apply in Northern Ireland.

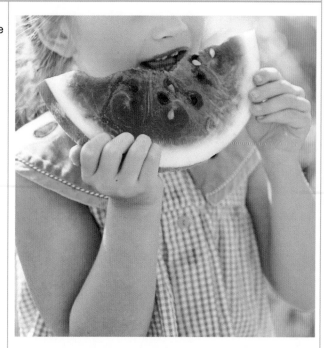

WHO SHOULD TAKE CHARGE OF THE PACK?

As a registered childminder / childcarer you should take charge of this pack.

CAN I USE SAFER FOOD, BETTER BUSINESS FOR CATERERS INSTEAD?

If you are already using Safer food, better business for caterers, you can continue using it if you prefer.

HOW DOES THE PACK WORK?

The pack contains eight 'safe method' sheets and a diary. The safe methods are divided into four different sections, each with a different colour and symbol.

The sections are named after 'the 4 Cs', which are the four main things to remember for good food hygiene: Cross-contamination, Cleaning, Chilling and Cooking. There is also a diary section.

CROSS-CONTAMINATION

Cross-contamination is one of the most common causes of food poisoning. It happens when harmful bacteria are spread onto food from other food, worktops, hands or equipment/utensils. These harmful bacteria often come from raw meat/poultry, fish, eggs and unwashed vegetables. Other sources of bacteria can include people, pests, pets, nappies and laundry.

Food also needs protecting from 'chemical contamination' (where chemicals get into food, e.g. cleaning products) and from 'physical contamination' (where objects get into food e.g. broken glass).

Good cleaning and handling practices can also help manage the risk of cross contamination from allergens.

CLEANING

Effective cleaning is essential to get rid of harmful bacteria and allergens, to stop them spreading to food.

CHILLING

Chilling food properly helps to stop harmful bacteria from growing. Some foods need to be kept chilled to keep them safe, such as foods with a 'use by' date. You also need to take care with frozen foods, especially when defrosting.

COOKING

It is essential to cook food properly to kill any harmful bacteria. If it is not cooked or reheated properly, it might not be safe for children or babies to eat. Some foods also need extra care, such as infant formula and breast milk.

DIARY

The diary is an important part of the pack. It helps you keep the records you need to comply with the law. The diary contains 'action sheets' and '3-monthly review' sheets. You can find out more about these under 'How to use the diary' below – and in the introduction to the diary section.

HOW TO USE THE SAFE METHODS

Front

The '**Safety point**' column highlights things that are important to make food safely.

Pictures help to illustrate the safety points.

The '**Why'?** column tells you why the safety point is important.

The '**How do you do this?**' column is for you to write down what you do.

In some places you only need to tick a box and in other places write a small amount.

SAFE METHOD:

KEEPING FOOD COLD

It is very important to keep certain foods cold because harmful bacteria can grow in them if they are not chilled properly. It is also important to take care when freezing or defrosting food.

SAFETY POINT	WHY?	HOW DO YOU DO THIS?
Certain foods need to be kept in the fridge to keep them safe e.g. • food with a 'use by' date • food that says 'keep refrigerated' on the label • cooked food e.g. food you have cooked in advance or leftovers • ready-to-eat food such as sandwiches, salads and some desserts Put food that you buy frozen e.g. ice cream, in the freezer straight away unless you are going to use it immediately.	If these types of food are not kept cold enough, harmful bacteria could grow.	Do you put these types of food into the fridge (or freezer) straight away? • When you return with shopping or when food is delivered? • when a parent/guardian brings food? • after you have used it? • after you have cooked and cooled down food? If not, what do you do?
Make sure that you do not use food after its 'use by' date.	Food that has passed its 'use by' date might not be safe to eat.	It is a good idea to check 'use by' dates every day.
Make sure your fridge is set at 5°C or below and your freezer is working properly. You should check the temperature of your fridge every day. You only need to write it down if something goes wrong.	Setting your fridge at 5°C will make sure the food is kept at 8°C or below. This is a legal requirement in England, Wales and Northern Ireland, and recommended in Scotland.	You can check this using a fridge thermometer. Some fridges will have a digital display to show what temperature they are set at but you should check regularly that the temperature shown on the display is accurate, using a fridge thermometer.
If you take food (e.g. sandwiches or yoghurts) with you when you go out, it is a good idea to use a cool bag and ice blocks to keep the food cold until you are ready to eat it.	It is important to keep chilled food cold to prevent harmful bacteria from growing.	Do you do this? Yes ☐ No ☐
If you cook food that will not be eaten immediately (or have leftovers), cool it down, ideally within one to two hours, and then put it in the fridge or freezer. Use up any leftovers within 48 hours. You can make food cool down more quickly by dividing food into smaller portions.	Harmful bacteria can grow in food if not cooled down quickly and then put in the fridge or freezer.	

Food Standards Agency | food.gov.uk/sfbb

An example of a completed safe method

Back

The '**What to do if things go wrong**' column gives practical tips on how to tackle problems.

If things go wrong, write down what happened and what you did in your action sheet. Each safe method reminds you to do this.

To complete the pack you need to work through each section and complete all the safe methods that are relevant to you. Fill in the date and sign each safe method when you have completed it.

Sometimes the pictures are marked with one of these symbols:

 RIGHT   WRONG

SAFETY POINTS	WHY?	HOW DO YOU DO THIS
Defrosting Food should be thoroughly defrosted before cooking (unless the manufacturer's instructions tell you to cook from frozen). If the manufacturer gives instructions on how to defrost the food, follow these.	If food is still frozen or partially frozen, it will take longer to cook. The outside of the food could be cooked, but the centre might not be, which means it could contain harmful bacteria.	Do you check food is thoroughly defrosted before cooking? Yes ☐ No ☐ If not, what do you do?
Ideally, defrost small amounts of food in the fridge. (Try to plan ahead and allow enough time for foods to defrost in this way.)	Putting food in the fridge will keep it at a safe temperature while it is defrosting.	Do you use this method? Yes
You could also defrost food in the microwave on the 'defrost' setting as long as the food is going to be cooked straight away.	This is a fast way to defrost food.	Do you use this method? Yes
Only defrost foods at room temperature if they do not need to be kept in the fridge e.g. bread.	Foods will defrost quite quickly at room temperature but harmful bacteria could grow in some food if it gets too warm while defrosting.	Do you use this method? Yes

THINK TWICE!

Once food has been defrosted keep it in the fridge and use it within 24 hours. Do not freeze the food again.

WHAT TO DO IF THINGS GO WRONG

• If you notice food has passed its 'use by' date, throw it away.
If your fridge is not working properly, you should:
• Move food that needs to be kept cold to another fridge (if you have one) or a cold area, or put it in a cool bag containing an ice block. If you cannot do this use the food straight away, or if you do not know how long the fridge has been broken down, throw the food away.
• If food that should be kept cold, has been left out of the fridge for a long time and is no longer cold, you should throw it away.
If you find that your freezer is not working properly, you should do the following things:
• If food is still frozen (i.e. hard and icy) it should be moved to another freezer straight away, if you have one.
• If you do not have another freezer, defrost the food safely and use it within 24 hours.
• If food has begun to defrost you should continue to defrost it safely and use within 24 hours.
• If food has fully defrosted (i.e. it is soft and warm), throw the food away.
• If food that needs to be kept frozen (e.g. ice cream) has started to defrost, do not refreeze it. Use it immediately or throw it away.

Write down what went wrong and what you did about it on your action sheet.

Safe method completed: Date:	Signature:

Food Standards Agency | food.gov.uk/sfbb

HOW TO USE THE DIARY

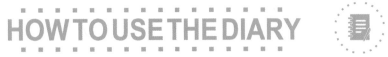

The diary includes action sheets and 3-monthly review sheets. These are an important part of the records you need to keep about food to comply with the law.

If you have any problems, or anything changes, you should make a note on the action sheet. Every three months, you should complete the 3-monthly review. See the introduction to the diary section for more information about this.

Fill in the date.

Write down what went wrong or what has changed.

Write down what you are going to do, or have already done, as a result.

Add your initials.

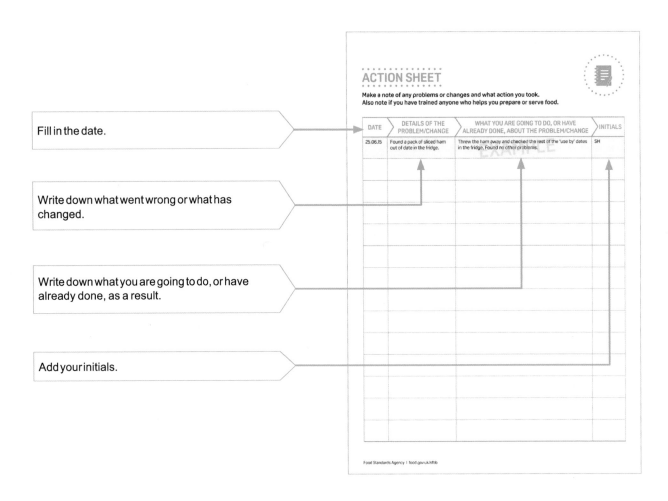

ACTION SHEET

Make a note of any problems or changes and what action you took.
Also note if you have trained anyone who helps you prepare or serve food.

DATE	DETAILS OF THE PROBLEM/CHANGE	WHAT YOU ARE GOING TO DO, OR HAVE ALREADY DONE, ABOUT THE PROBLEM/CHANGE	INITIALS
25.06.15	Found a pack of sliced ham out of date in the fridge.	Threw the ham away and checked the rest of the 'use by' dates in the fridge. Found no other problems.	SH

Food Standards Agency | food.gov.uk/sfbb

HOW TO USE THE DIARY

Fill in the date.

Tick to say you have completed your 3-monthly review.

Write down details of any serious or persistent problems and any changes in the way you are working.

Give details of any action you are going to take, or have already taken, as a result of the problem / change. Also write down any changes you need to make to your safe methods.

3-MONTHLY REVIEW

The 3-monthly review is an important part of the records you need to keep about food to comply with the law.

Every three months you should look back at previous months and identify any problems. If you had a serious or persistent problem (the same thing went wrong three times or more), make a note of it below and also write down what you are going to do, or have already done, about it.

There might also have been changes in the way you are working with food e.g:
• Have you changed the ingredients, types of food or recipes you use?
• Are you looking after a new child? Do they have any allergies or need different foods?
• Are you using any different equipment?

If there have been any changes like these, you will need to review your safe methods to make sure they are up to date. Make a note of what has changed below and give details of any changes you need to make to your safe methods.

If you need a new copy of a safe method, you can download one from **food.gov.uk/childminders**. Remember to sign and date the safe method after you have filled it in.

DATE	3-MONTHLY REVIEW COMPLETED	DETAILS OF A SERIOUS OR PERSISTENT PROBLEM OR A CHANGE IN THE WAY YOU ARE WORKING	WHAT YOU ARE GOING TO DO, OR HAVE ALREADY DONE, ABOUT THE PROBLEM OR ANY CHANGES YOU NEED TO MAKE TO YOUR SAFE METHODS
25.06.15	✓	Have a new baby in my care (Richard Brown).	Need to change the 'Babies and children – special advice' safe method to show how I store made-up formula milk provided by the parents.
25.06.15	✓	No problem / changes	No action to take
	☐		
	☐		

EXAMPLE

Food Standards Agency | food.gov.uk/sfbb

WHAT DO I DO NEXT?

Work through the pack and fill in all of the safe methods that are relevant to you.

Most childminders will need to fill in all the safe methods. But if, for example, you only serve cold food e.g. sandwiches, then the 'Cooking and reheating' safe method would not be relevant.

Remember that once you have worked through the pack, you need to make sure you are following the safe methods every day.

DO I NEED TO KEEP LOTS OF DAILY RECORDS?

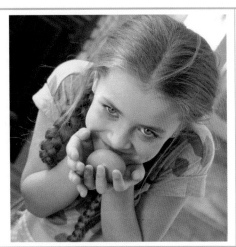

No, you will not need to keep lots of daily records. Once you have worked through the pack and filled in all of the relevant safe methods, you will only need to fill in the action sheet if you have a problem or something changes, and to complete the 3-monthly review. See the 'How to use the diary' section for more information.

It is a legal requirement to keep a record of what food products you have bought, who you bought them from, the quantity and date. Usually the easiest way to do this is to keep all your receipts, even for small amounts. This is so that – if there is a safety problem with food you have provided – you or an enforcement officer from your local authority can check the details of the food.

Keep these records in a way that makes it easy for you or an enforcement officer to check them. There is no set time for how long you need to keep these but as a guide keep them until you are sure the food they refer to has been consumed by the children, without any problem.

WHAT IF I NEED EXTRA COPIES OF THE SAFE METHODS OR DIARY PAGES?

If you need a new copy of a safe method, you can download one from **food.gov.uk/childminders**. If you need more copies of the action sheet or the 3-monthly review sheet, you can either download them or photocopy the sheets in the pack before you have filled them in.

DOES ANYONE ELSE NEED TO USE THIS PACK?

If anyone helps you to prepare or serve food for the children / babies you look after, it is very important to train them in all the safe methods that are relevant to what they do. Make sure they have worked through the 'Personal hygiene' safe method before they do any work with food. You should also supervise them to check they are following the safe methods properly. Keep a note of any training on the action sheet in your diary.

WHERE CAN I GET MORE INFORMATION?

For more information about food safety, talk to the environmental health department at your local authority or visit **food.gov.uk/business-industry/caterers/startingup/childminders**

For details of Food Standards Agency publications visit **food.gov.uk/publications**

For more information about what foods to give to babies and children, see **http://www.nhs.uk/Conditions/pregnancy-and-baby/pages/understanding-food-groups.aspx#close**

England – you can find more information on registration as a childminder or childcarer on domestic premises on the Ofsted website at **www.ofsted.gov.uk**

Scotland – visit the Care Inspectorate at **www.careinspectorate.com**

Wales – visit the Care and Social Services Inspectorate Wales at **www.cssiw.org.uk**

Northern Ireland – contact the Early Years team at your local Health and Social Services Trust.

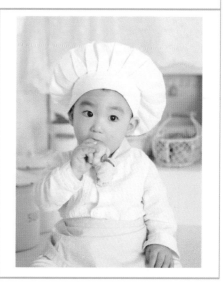

ABOUT THIS GUIDANCE

This guidance follows the Government Code of Practice on Guidance. If you believe this guidance breaches the Code for any reason, or if you have any comments on the guidance, please contact us at **FoodBusinessHygiene@foodstandards.gsi.gov.uk**

This guidance was originally published in 2009. The most recent update is December 2015 and it will be reviewed again in December 2018.

COPYRIGHT

PERSONAL HYGIENE

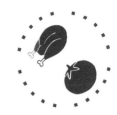

It is important to follow good personal hygiene to help prevent bacteria from spreading to food.

SAFETY POINT	WHY?
Avoid touching your face or nose, or coughing and sneezing over food.	Harmful bacteria and viruses can be spread from your face, nose or mouth to your hands and onto food.
Ideally you should not wear watches or jewellery when preparing food (except a plain wedding band).	Watches and jewellery can collect and spread dirt and harmful bacteria and fall in the food.
Make sure your clothes are clean and ideally wear an apron when preparing food.	Clothes can bring dirt and bacteria into food preparation areas. Wearing clean clothes helps to prevent this.
Do not prepare any food if you have diarrhoea and / or vomiting.	People suffering from these symptoms often carry harmful bacteria and viruses on their hands and can spread them to food or equipment they touch.
Do not prepare food until you have had no symptoms for 48 hours.	Even if the diarrhoea and vomiting has stopped, you can still carry harmful bacteria for 48 hours afterwards.
Cuts and sores should be completely covered with a waterproof dressing, ideally a brightly coloured one.	This is to prevent bacteria from the cut or sore spreading to food. Brightly coloured dressings are easier to spot if they come off and fall into food.

HANDWASHING

SAFETY POINT	WHY?
You should always wash your hands properly before preparing and handling food or touching ready-to-eat food e.g. sandwiches. You should wash your hands after: • going to the toilet • touching raw meat / poultry, fish, eggs and unwashed vegetables • emptying bins • cleaning • touching a cut or changing a dressing • handling pets, their feeding bowls or other equipment • contact with potties, nappies and changing mats • cleaning up accidents (e.g. vomit or diarrhoea) • helping a child use the toilet • wiping or blowing your nose or a child's nose • outside activities e.g. after taking children to the park • touching dirty laundry	Harmful bacteria can spread very easily from hands to food, work surfaces and equipment. Washing your hands properly at the right times helps to prevent this. 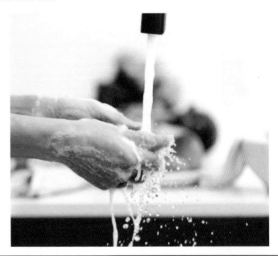

WASHING HANDS EFFECTIVELY

Step 1:

Wet your hands thoroughly under warm running water and squirt liquid soap onto your palm.

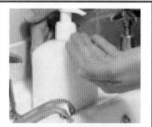

Step 2:

Rub your hands together palm to palm to make a lather.

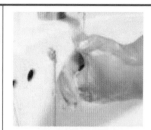

Step 3:

Rub the palm of one hand along the back of the other and along the fingers. Repeat with the other hand.

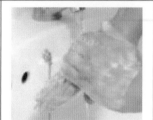

Step 4:

Put your palms together with fingers interlocked and rub in between each of the fingers thoroughly, and around the fingertips and thumbs.

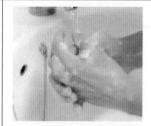

Step 5:

Rinse off the soap with clean water.

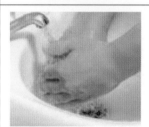

Step 6:

Dry hands thoroughly with a clean towel that you only use for drying hands.

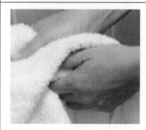

THINK TWICE!

- Make sure anyone else who prepares food for the children, or uses the kitchen, understands the importance of personal hygiene, and especially the importance of washing hands properly. Harmful bacteria can spread very easily from people's hands to food, work surfaces, equipment etc. Effective handwashing helps to prevent this.
- Make sure children wash their hands before eating.
- Make sure you have a good supply of soap and clean towels for handwashing.

WHAT TO DO IF THINGS GO WRONG

If you think someone who is helping you has not washed their hands, make sure they wash them straight away and emphasise how important it is to wash their hands when working with food.

Write down what went wrong and what you did about it in your action sheet.

Safe method completed: Date: [   ]   Signature: [   ]

FOOD STORAGE AND PREPARATION

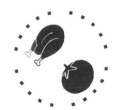

It is very important to store and prepare food carefully and keep sources of bacteria and allergens away from food preparation areas.

SAFETY POINT >	WHY? >	HOW DO YOU DO THIS?
Ideally, store raw and ready-to-eat food separately. If they are in the same fridge, store raw meat and poultry, fish and eggs below ready-to-eat food, such as salads, sandwiches and desserts. Unwashed fruit and vegetables should also be kept separate from ready-to-eat food and above raw meat. If you are defrosting raw meat or poultry, make sure that none of the liquid that comes out of it gets onto other food. Cover cooked and other ready-to-eat food. Keep food that contains allergens separate from other food.	This helps to prevent harmful bacteria spreading from raw food to ready-to-eat food. 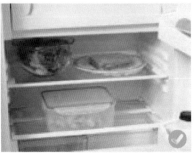 This will stop allergens from spreading.	Do you store raw meat and poultry? Yes ☐ No ☐ If yes, do you follow this advice? Yes ☐ If not, what do you do?
Never use the same worktop, chopping board, knives or other equipment for preparing raw food (such as meat and poultry) and for ready-to-eat food, unless they have been thoroughly cleaned and disinfected in between. See the 'Cleaning' safe method.	Harmful bacteria from raw food such as meat/poultry can spread from chopping boards and knives to other food. 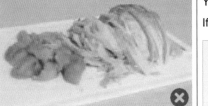	Do you always use a clean knife and chopping board for preparing ready-to-eat food? Yes ☐ If not, what do you do?
Do not wash raw meat or poultry.	Washing meat and poultry does not kill bacteria but it can splash harmful bacteria around the kitchen, contaminating sinks, taps, surfaces and ready-to-eat food.	More information can be found at: **food.gov.uk/news-updates/campaigns/campylobacter/actnow**
When preparing fruit, vegetables and salad ingredients wash them thoroughly by rubbing vigorously in a bowl of clean water. Wash the cleanest ones first.	Fruit, vegetables and salad ingredients may have harmful bacteria on the outside. Washing will help clean them and remove some of the bacteria.	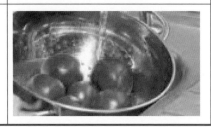

'USE BY' AND 'BEST BEFORE' DATES – WHAT THEY MEAN

'Use by' date – this is about safety. Do not serve food after this date – this is against the law. Even if it looks and smells fine, eating food after its 'use by' date could make children or babies ill.

'Best before' date – this is about quality. Food should be safe to eat after the 'best before' date, but it might begin to lose its flavour and texture. Eggs are an exception – they should always be used by their 'best before' date.

SAFETY POINT	WHY?	HOW DO YOU DO THIS?

Nappies and laundry

If your washing machine is in the kitchen, do not bring dirty laundry into the kitchen while food is being prepared.

Your nappy changing facilities should be separate from any food preparation areas.

Never put dirty nappies, laundry or laundry baskets on worktops.

Always wash your hands properly after touching dirty nappies or laundry.

This helps to prevent dirt and bacteria spreading from nappies and laundry to food.

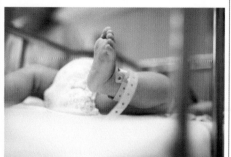

If your washing machine is in the kitchen, do you follow this advice?

Yes ☐   No ☐

If not what do you do?

Where are your nappy changing facilities?

Pets

Keep pets away from all food, dishes and worktops and away from children when they are eating.

If pets have access to the kitchen, clean and disinfect worktops before you start food preparation.

Pets can spread harmful bacteria to food.

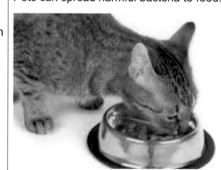

Do you have any pets?

Yes ☐   No ☐

If yes, do you follow this advice?

Yes ☐

If not, what do you do?

SAFETY POINT	WHY?

Maintenance

Make sure you keep food preparation areas in good condition.

Replace damaged equipment, utensils and dishes straight away e.g. replace worn chopping boards, cracked dishes, chipped glasses.

This makes cleaning easier and helps to prevent pests.

Dirt and bacteria can collect on damaged equipment/utensils and loose parts might fall into food.

WHAT TO DO IF THINGS GO WRONG

- If raw meat / poultry, fish, eggs or unwashed vegetables have touched or dripped onto ready-to-eat or cooked food, throw away the food.

- If ready-to-eat or cooked food has been prepared using a worktop, chopping board, knife or other equipment that has been used with raw food and not cleaned and disinfected afterwards, throw away the food.

- If dirty laundry, nappies or pets have been on a worktop, remove them and wash and then disinfect the worktop straight away.

- If there is a risk that an object (such as broken glass) may have got into food, throw the food away.

Write down what went wrong and what you did about it in your action sheet.

Safe method completed: Date: _____	Signature:	

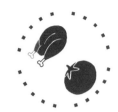

FOOD ALLERGIES

It is important to know what to do if you look after a child who has a food allergy, because these allergies can be life-threatening

SAFETY POINT	WHY?
Always check if children have any food allergies and keep a written record of these.	It is a good idea to be able to refer to this record when preparing and serving food.
Make sure you check all the ingredients of any meals and snacks you give to a child with a food allergy. For example, if you make a cheese sandwich, check the ingredients of the bread, cheese, spread and anything else you put in the sandwich. **Never guess**.	If someone has a severe allergy, they can react to even a tiny amount of the food they are sensitive to. You can find out more about allergies at **food.gov.uk/ business-industry/allergy-guide**
Keep a record of the ingredient information of any ready-made food and drink you use in the children's food. Separating and labelling ingredients is very important to help you to easily identify what is in the meal.	This is so you can check what is in the food.
If you are cooking, remember to check the ingredients of any oil, sauce, dressing or other packaged foods, including tins and jars. If you are not sure, do not give the food to the child.	Any of these could contain an ingredient the child is allergic to.
When you are preparing food for a child with a food allergy, clean worktops and equipment thoroughly before you start. Make sure you also wash your hands thoroughly first.	This is to prevent small amounts of the food that a child is allergic to getting into the food by accident.
If a parent / guardian of a child with an allergy provides food, make sure it is clearly labelled with the child's name.	This makes sure that the child receives the right food and avoids it being given to another child who may have a different food allergy.

HOW DO YOU DO THIS?

How do you check if food does not contain a particular allergen / ingredient?

How do you prepare food for a child with a food allergy?

THINK TWICE!

Which ingredients can cause a problem?

If asked, you must provide information about the allergens (if they are used as ingredients in the food and drink you provide) to the parents / carers of the children in your care. You can find further information here: **food.gov.uk/business-industry/ caterers/startingup/childminders**

These are some of the foods children may be allergic to and where they may be found:

Nuts (Namely almonds, hazelnuts, walnuts, pecan nuts, Brazil nuts, pistachio, cashew, Macadamia or Queensland nut).	In sauces, desserts, crackers, bread, ice cream, marzipan, ground almonds, nut oils.
Peanuts	In sauces, cakes, desserts. Don't forget groundnut oil and peanut flour.
Eggs	In cakes, mousses, sauces, pasta, quiche, some meat products. Don't forget foods containing mayonnaise or brushed with egg.
Milk	In yoghurt, cream, cheese, butter, milk powders. Also check for foods glazed with milk.
Fish	In some salad dressings, pizzas, relishes, fish sauce. You might also find fish in some soy and Worcestershire sauces.
Crustaceans	Such as prawns, lobster, scampi, crab, shrimp paste.
Molluscs	These include mussels, whelks, squid, land snails, oyster sauce.
Cereals containing gluten (namely wheat (such as spelt and Khorasan wheat), barley, rye and oats)	Also check foods containing flour, such as bread, pasta, cakes, pastry, meat products, sauces, soups, batter, stock cubes, breadcrumbs, foods dusted with flour.
Celery	This includes celery stalks, leaves and seeds and celeriac. Also look out for celery in salads, soups, celery salt, some meat products.
Lupin	Lupin seeds and flour in some types of bread and pastries.
Mustard	Including liquid mustard, mustard powder and mustard seeds, in salad dressings, marinades, soups, sauces, curries, meat products.
Sesame seeds	In bread, breadsticks, tahini, houmous, sesame oil.
Soya	As tofu or beancurd, soya flour and textured soya protein, in some ice cream, sauces, desserts, meat products, vegetarian products.
Sulphur dioxide (when added and above 10mg / kg in the finished food and drink)	In meat products, fruit juice drinks, dried fruit and vegetables, wine, beer.

WHAT TO DO IF THINGS GO WRONG 〉 HOW TO STOP THIS HAPPENING AGAIN

WHAT TO DO IF THINGS GO WRONG	HOW TO STOP THIS HAPPENING AGAIN
If you think a child is having a severe allergic reaction: • Do not move them • If the child has a prescribed adrenaline auto-injector e.g. Epi pen and you have been trained to use it, administer it according to the child's care plan. • Ring 999 and ask for an ambulance with a paramedic straight away • Explain that the child could have anaphylaxis (pronounced 'anna-fill-axis') • Send a responsible person outside to wait for the ambulance • Contact the parent / guardian of the child after you have called an ambulance.	• Make sure that you and anyone who helps with food preparation, understands how important it is to check all the ingredients of a food and knows about the symptoms and treatment of an allergic reaction. You can find out more about this at **nhs.uk/conditions/pregnancy-and-baby/pages/food-allergies-in-children.aspx#close** • Review the way food is prepared for a child with a food allergy – are you cleaning effectively first and using clean equipment?

Safe method completed: Date: _____ Signature: _____

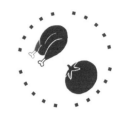

PEST CONTROL AND CHEMICAL CONTAMINATION

Effective pest control is essential to keep out pests and prevent them from spreading harmful bacteria. It is also very important that you prevent chemicals getting into food.

SAFETY POINT	WHY?
Pests	
Check regularly for signs of pests, for example, in your food cupboards.	Pests can carry harmful bacteria.
Make sure no food or dirty plates are left out at night. And clean up any food on the floor.	These are a source of food for pests.

TYPES OF PESTS

Rats and mice Look out for droppings, gnawed food or packaging. 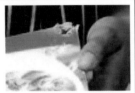	**Cockroaches and ants** Look out for the insects themselves.	**Flies and other insects** Look out for insects and maggots. 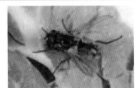

SAFETY POINT	WHY?
Chemicals	
Always read the label and follow the manufacturer's instructions on how to use chemicals.	This is important to make sure that chemicals work effectively.
Never let pest control bait / chemicals, including sprays, come into contact with food, packaging, equipment or worktops.	Chemicals are likely to be poisonous to people.
Store cleaning chemicals (e.g. bleach, detergents) separately from food and make sure they are clearly labelled.	Storing chemicals properly is very important to keep food and children safe.
Keep all cleaning and pest control products out of reach of children.	

WHAT TO DO IF THINGS GO WRONG

- If you see signs of pests, call your local authority or a pest contractor immediately.
- If you think any equipment, worktops or utensils have been touched by pests, wash and then disinfect them thoroughly to stop harmful bacteria from spreading.
- If you think food has been touched by pests in any way, throw it away.
- If there is a risk that pest control or cleaning chemicals may have got into food, throw the food away.

Write down what went wrong and what you did about it in your action sheet.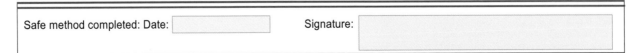

Safe method completed: Date: _____ Signature: _____

CLEANING

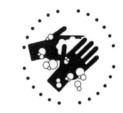

It is essential to keep your food preparation areas clean to get rid of harmful bacteria and allergens to stop them spreading.

SAFETY POINT	WHY?
Regularly clean and disinfect all the items people touch frequently, such as worktops, sinks, taps, handles, switches and high chairs. Cleaning needs to be carried out in two stages. First use a cleaning product to remove visible dirt from surfaces and equipment, and rinse. Then disinfect them following the manufacturers instructions and rinse with fresh clean water. If you use an all-in-one spray this should be used first to clean and again to disinfect. Allow these items to dry naturally or dry them with disposable kitchen towel.	It is important to keep these items clean to prevent dirt, harmful bacteria and allergens being spread to people's hands and then from their hands to food or other areas. 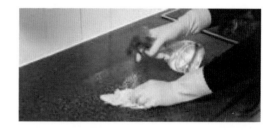
Wash worktops, chopping boards and knives thoroughly before preparing food. Wash and disinfect them after preparing raw meat / poultry, fish, eggs or unwashed vegetables. Ideally, wash them in a dishwasher, if appropriate. Do not overload the dishwasher and make sure it is maintained and serviced regularly. If you do not have a dishwasher, wash them in hot soapy water using diluted detergent. Remove grease and any food and dirt, then immerse them in very hot, clean water. Leave to air dry, or dry with a disposable kitchen towel. Wipe up any spills as soon as they happen. Clean and then disinfect after wiping up spills from raw food.	This will help prevent dirt and harmful bacteria spreading onto food from the surface or equipment. Dishwashers wash items thoroughly at a high temperature, so this is a good way to clean equipment and kill bacteria (disinfect) and remove allergens.
Always use a clean cloth to wipe worktops, equipment or utensils. Ideally, use disposable kitchen towel wherever possible. Make sure cloths are thoroughly washed, disinfected and dried between tasks (not just when they look dirty). It is important to also wash and disinfect tea towels and oven gloves regularly. Ideally, wash cloths, tea towels, aprons and oven gloves separately from other laundry, in a washing machine on a hot cycle of 90°C. This will disinfect them. Or if you wash them by hand, make sure all the food and dirt has been removed by washing in hot soapy water before disinfecting them with very hot clean water.	Using dirty cloths or tea towels can spread harmful bacteria or allergens very easily. Using disposable kitchen towel will make sure that any bacteria or allergens picked up on the towel will not be spread. 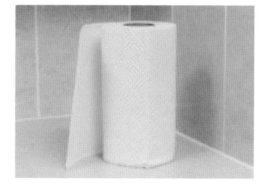

SAFETY POINT	WHY?
When cleaning up accidents (e.g. vomiting or diarrhoea) make sure that you clean, wash and disinfect the area thoroughly.	This prevents harmful bacteria from spreading.
Do not allow kitchen cloths to be used elsewhere in the house, e.g. when cleaning up after accidents (vomit or diarrhoea).	This is to prevent harmful bacteria spreading to the kitchen.
Follow the manufacturer's instructions on how to use and store cleaning chemicals. When you clean worktops / chopping boards, make sure that any cleaning chemicals you use are suitable for surfaces touched by food. Keep all chemicals out of reach of children.	Using and storing chemicals correctly is important to make sure they are effective and to keep children and food safe.

WHAT TO DO IF THINGS GO WRONG

- If you find that any item in your kitchen is not properly clean, wash and disinfect it and allow it to dry.
- If you think that a kitchen cloth has been used elsewhere in the house, throw the cloth away or wash and disinfect it before you use it again.
- After cleaning up accidents, change your clothes if you need to and make sure you wash your hands properly afterwards.

Write down what went wrong and what you did about it on your action sheet

Safe method completed: Date: [   ]   Signature: [   ]

KEEPING FOOD COLD

It is very important to keep certain foods cold because harmful bacteria can grow in them if they are not chilled properly. It is also important to take care when freezing or defrosting food.

SAFETY POINT	WHY?	HOW DO YOU DO THIS?
Certain foods need to be kept in the fridge to keep them safe e.g. • food with a 'use by' date • food that says 'keep refrigerated' on the label • cooked food e.g. food you have cooked in advance or leftovers • ready-to-eat food such as sandwiches, salads, cooked meat and some desserts Put food that you buy frozen e.g. ice cream, in the freezer straight away unless you are going to use it immediately.	If these types of food are not kept cold enough, harmful bacteria could grow.	Do you put these types of food into the fridge (or freezer) straight away: • When you return with shopping or when food is delivered? ☐ • when a parent / guardian brings food? ☐ • after you have used it? ☐ • after you have cooked and cooled down food? ☐ If not, what do you do?
Make sure that you do not use food after its 'use by' date.	Food that has passed its 'use by' date might not be safe to eat.	It is a good idea to check 'use by' dates every day.
Make sure your fridge is set at 5°C or below and your freezer is working properly. You should check the temperature of your fridge every day. You only need to write it down if something goes wrong.	Setting your fridge at 5°C will make sure the food is kept at 8°C or below. This is a legal requirement in England, Wales and Northern Ireland, and recommended in Scotland.	You can check this using a fridge thermometer. Some fridges will have a digital display to show what temperature they are set at but you should check regularly that the temperature shown on the display is accurate, using a fridge thermometer.
If you take food (e.g. sandwiches or yoghurts) with you when you go out, it is a good idea to use a cool bag and ice blocks to keep the food cold until you are ready to eat it.	It is important to keep chilled food cold to prevent harmful bacteria from growing.	Do you do this? Yes ☐ No ☐
If you cook food that will not be eaten immediately (or have leftovers), cool it down, ideally within one to two hours, and then put it in the fridge or freezer. Use up any leftovers within 48 hours. You can make food cool down more quickly by dividing food into smaller portions.	Harmful bacteria can grow in food if not cooled down quickly and then put in the fridge or freezer.	

SAFETY POINTS	WHY?	HOW DO YOU DO THIS
Defrosting Food should be thoroughly defrosted before cooking (unless the manufacturer's instructions tell you to cook from frozen). If the manufacturer gives instructions on how to defrost the food, follow these.	If food is still frozen or partially frozen, it will take longer to cook. The outside of the food could be cooked, but the centre might not be, which means it could contain harmful bacteria.	Do you check food is thoroughly defrosted before cooking? Yes ☐ No ☐ If not, what do you do?
Ideally, defrost small amounts of food in the fridge. (Try to plan ahead and allow enough time for foods to defrost in this way.)	Putting food in the fridge will keep it at a safe temperature while it is defrosting.	Do you use this method? Yes ☐
You could also defrost food in the microwave on the 'defrost' setting as long as the food is going to be cooked straight away.	This is a fast way to defrost food.	Do you use this method? Yes ☐
Only defrost foods at room temperature if they do not need to be kept in the fridge e.g. bread.	Foods will defrost quite quickly at room temperature but harmful bacteria could grow in some food if it gets too warm while defrosting.	Do you do this? Yes ☐ No ☐

THINK TWICE!

Keep meat / poultry separate from other food when it is defrosting, to prevent cross-contamination. Once food has been defrosted keep it in the fridge and use it within 24 hours. Do not freeze the food again.

WHAT TO DO IF THINGS GO WRONG

- If you notice food has passed its 'use by' date, throw it away.

If your fridge is not working properly, you should:

- Move food that needs to be kept cold to another fridge (if you have one) or a cold area, or put it in a cool bag containing an ice block. If you cannot do this use the food straight away, or if you do not know how long the fridge has been broken down, throw the food away.
- If food that should be kept cold, has been left out of the fridge for a long time and is no longer cold, you should throw it away.

If you find that your freezer is not working properly, you should do the following things:

- **If food is still frozen** (i.e. hard and icy) it should be moved to another freezer straight away, if you have one. If you do not have another freezer, defrost the food safely and use within 24 hours.
- **If food has begun to defrost** you should continue to defrost it safely and use within 24 hours.
- **If food has fully defrosted** (i.e. it is soft and warm), throw the food away.
- **If food that needs to be kept frozen** (e.g. ice cream) has started to defrost, do not refreeze it. Use it immediately or throw it away.

Write down what went wrong and what you did about it on your action sheet

Safe method completed: Date:	Signature:

COOKING AND REHEATING SAFELY

Thorough cooking kills harmful bacteria. It is also very important to reheat food properly to kill harmful bacteria that may have grown since the food was cooked.

SAFETY POINT	WHY?
If a food has manufacturer's cooking instructions, follow these. Always check that food is very hot (steaming) all the way through. You can also use the following checks to make sure that food is properly cooked or reheated.	The manufacturer has tried and tested safe cooking methods specifically for its products.

TYPES OF CHECK	TYPES OF FOOD
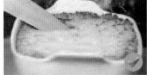 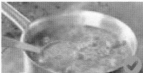 Check that food you are cooking or reheating is very hot (steaming) all the way through. Check the centre of dishes such as shepherd's pie or lasagne.	**Circle the types of food you use this check for and add any others.** **Types of food:** stew, curry, soup, gravy, pasta dishes, fish, rice, pies and pasties, fish fingers, pizzas, stir fries. **Other foods:**
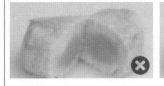 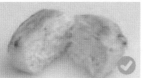 Check that pieces of chicken are very hot (steaming) in the middle. The meat should not be pink or red and the juices should not have any pink or red in them. If you are cooking a whole chicken, check the meat in the thickest part of the leg.	**Types of food:** chicken drumstick and leg, chicken curry, chicken nuggets. **Other foods:**
Check that pork, liver and processed meat products, such as sausages and burgers, are very hot (steaming) all the way through with no pink or red in the centre. 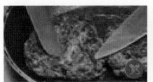 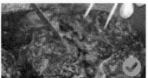	**Types of food:** burgers, sausages, meatballs, pork chops, liver, gammon. **Other foods:**
Check that all the outside surfaces of meat are fully cooked. 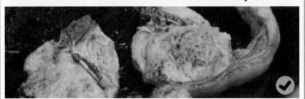	**Types of food:** lamb chops, lamb cutlets, steak, joints of beef and lamb. **Other foods:**

TYPES OF CHECK	TYPES OF FOOD

Eggs

Do not serve raw eggs or make foods with raw or partially cooked eggs (e.g. home-made mayonnaise, mousse or ice cream) because these can contain harmful bacteria. Do not let children taste cake mixture containing raw eggs.

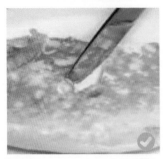

Avoid giving eggs with runny yolks to babies and toddlers.

For other egg dishes and foods containing eggs e.g. scrambled eggs, omelettes and quiche, check they are very hot (steaming) all the way through.

Do not use eggs after the 'best before' date. After this date there is a greater chance of harmful bacteria growing in the eggs. Ideally keep eggs in the fridge.

Do you cook egg dishes and foods containing eggs thoroughly until they are very hot (steaming)?

Yes ☐ No ☐

If not, what do you do?

Rice

When you have cooked rice, make sure you keep it hot until it is eaten or cool it down as quickly as possible (ideally within one hour) and then keep it in the fridge. Use cooked rice within 24 hours and reheat it until very hot (steaming).

Rice can contain spores from a type of harmful bacteria. If cooked rice is left at room temperature, the bacteria could start growing again from the spores. These bacteria will multiply and may produce toxins (poisons) that cause food poisoning. Reheating will not get rid of these.

Do you either keep rice hot or cool it down as quickly as possible and keep it in the fridge?

Yes ☐ No ☐

If not, what do you do?

THINK TWICE!

Reheating

Remember, reheating means cooking again, not just warming up. To make sure that cooked or reheated food is safe to eat, always check it is very hot (steaming) all the way through and then, if you need to, let it cool a little before serving it to a child. You should only reheat food once.

If you are reheating food in a microwave, follow the product manufacturer's instructions, if you have them, including advice on standing and stirring. Standing and stirring are part of the process of cooking / reheating in a microwave and help to make sure that food is the same temperature all the way through.

If you use a microwave to reheat food that you, or a parent / carer have cooked, it is a good idea to stir it while reheating. When food is microwaved, it can be very hot at the edges and still be cold in the centre – stirring helps to prevent this.

WHAT TO DO IF THINGS GO WRONG

- If food is not properly cooked or reheated, cook it for longer.
- Speed up the cooking process, for example by dividing the food into smaller quantities, or using different equipment.
- Check that your oven / hob / microwave is working properly.

Write down what went wrong and what you did about it in your action sheet.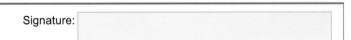

Safe method completed: Date:	Signature:

BABIES AND CHILDREN – SPECIAL ADVICE

There are some foods for babies that need extra care and others that are not suitable for children.

SAFETY POINT	WHY?	HOW DO YOU DO THIS?
Formula milk If parents / carers bring made-up bottles of formula, put them in the fridge straight away. Keep them in the fridge until you are ready to use them. Use the formula within 24 hours. Before you prepare a feed, clean worktops and wash your hands. You should clean and sterilise bottles and teats before you use them. Follow the manufacturer's instructions on how to do this. For more information on sterilising bottles, go to **nhs.uk/conditions/ pregnancy-and-baby/pages/ sterilising-bottles.aspx#close**	If formula is not used as soon as it has been made up, it needs to be kept cold to help keep it safe. Making sure that everything is clean reduces the chance of a baby getting sickness and diarrhoea.	Do you do this? Yes ☐ No ☐ If not, what do you do?
Ideally, you should make up formula milk freshly for each feed. If there is any made-up formula milk left after a feed, throw it away. Boil fresh tap water and let it cool, but for no more than half an hour. Always put the boiled water in the bottle first, before the powder. Cool the formula quickly to feeding temperature by holding the bottle under cold running water (with the cap on).	Using made-up formula milk that has been stored may increase the chance of a baby becoming ill. Using hot water will kill any harmful bacteria in the powder.	Do you do this? Yes ☐ No ☐ If not, what do you do?
Breast milk Expressed breast milk should be stored in the fridge and used within 24 hours.	If expressed milk is not kept cold, harmful bacteria may grow in it.	

SAFETY POINT	WHY?
Baby food If you are using bought baby food, follow the manufacturer's instructions on how to prepare and serve it. If you make your own baby food (or a parent / carer brings home-made baby food), it is very important to cook, cool, store, defrost and reheat it safely. Follow the advice in the 'Keeping food cold' and 'Cooking and reheating safely' safe methods.	The manufacturer will have designed its instructions to make sure the food is safe for babies to eat. If you do not handle baby food safely, harmful bacteria could grow in the food.
Honey Do not give honey to children under one year old. 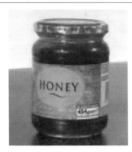	Very occasionally, honey can contain a type of harmful bacteria that can produce toxins in a baby's intestines and this can cause serious illness.
Fish Do not give shark, swordfish and marlin to babies and young children.	These fish contain relatively high levels of mercury, which might affect a child's developing nervous system.
Shellfish Avoid giving raw shellfish to babies and young children.	Raw shellfish can contain harmful viruses and bacteria.
Nuts Do not give whole nuts to children under five. It is a good idea to crush or flake them.	This is because of the risk of choking.

For more advice on what foods to give to babies and children, visit **www.nhs.uk/Conditions/pregnancy-andbaby/pages/pregnancy-and-baby-care.aspx**

Safe method completed: Date: Signature:

INTRODUCTION

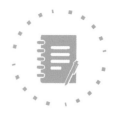

WHAT IS IN THIS DIARY SECTION?

The diary includes:

- action sheets
- 3-monthly review sheets

These are an important part of the records you need to keep about food to comply with the law. An environmental health officer from your local authority may want to check these if they visit you.

If you need more copies of the action sheet or the 3-monthly review sheet, you can either download them from **food.gov.uk/ childminders** or photocopy the sheets in the pack before you have filled them in.

WHAT DO I NEED TO DO?

This pack has been designed to involve as little paperwork as possible. That means that, once you have worked through the pack and you are following your safe methods, you do not have to write anything down, unless there has been a problem, or something has changed – or it is time for your 3-monthly review.

If there are any problems or changes, fill in the action sheet to give details of the problem / change and what you are going to do, or have already done, about it.

HOW TO COMPLETE THE 3-MONTHLY REVIEW

Every three months you should look back at previous months and identify any serious or persistent problems, or any changes in the way you are working. You may need to take action to solve a problem, or make changes to your safe methods. Fill in the details on the 3-monthly review sheet.

If you notice a recurring problem before the 3-monthly review is due, you should always take action at the time to resolve it, rather than waiting until the next review. Make a note of what you have done on your action sheet.

Some childminders might prefer to keep more records than required by this pack – that is fine, but make sure you still use the action sheet and 3-monthly review.

CHANGING A SAFE METHOD

Sometimes you might need to change one of your safe methods because of a problem or a change in the way you are working. If you can, change the current copy of the safe method so it is still clear to read, then add the date of the change at the bottom and also make a note on your action sheet.

Sometimes you might need a new copy of a safe method (you can download this from **food.gov.uk/childminders**). Sign and date it at the bottom when you have filled it in and keep it in your pack. You can throw away the old copy of the safe method. Don't forget to make a note of what you have done on your action sheet.

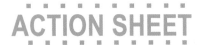

ACTION SHEET

Make a note of any problems or changes and what action you took.
Also note if you have trained anyone who helps you prepare or serve food.

DATE	DETAILS OF THE PROBLEM / CHANGE	WHAT YOU ARE GOING TO DO, OR HAVE ALREADY DONE, ABOUT THE PROBLEM / CHANGE	INITIALS
25.06.15	Found a pack of sliced ham out of date in the fridge.	Threw the ham away and checked the rest of the 'use by' dates in the fridge. Found no other problems.	SH

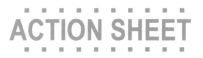

ACTION SHEET

DATE	DETAILS OF THE PROBLEM/CHANGE	WHAT YOU ARE GOING TO DO, OR HAVE ALREADY DONE, ABOUT THE PROBLEM/CHANGE	INITIALS

ACTION SHEET

DATE	DETAILS OF THE PROBLEM/CHANGE	WHAT YOU ARE GOING TO DO, OR HAVE ALREADY DONE, ABOUT THE PROBLEM/CHANGE	INITIALS

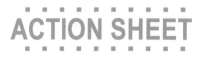

ACTION SHEET

DATE	DETAILS OF THE PROBLEM/CHANGE	WHAT YOU ARE GOING TO DO, OR HAVE ALREADY DONE, ABOUT THE PROBLEM/CHANGE	INITIALS

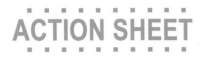

ACTION SHEET

DATE	DETAILS OF THE PROBLEM/CHANGE	WHAT YOU ARE GOING TO DO, OR HAVE ALREADY DONE, ABOUT THE PROBLEM/CHANGE	INITIALS

ACTION SHEET

DATE	DETAILS OF THE PROBLEM/CHANGE	WHAT YOU ARE GOING TO DO, OR HAVE ALREADY DONE, ABOUT THE PROBLEM/CHANGE	INITIALS

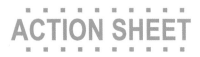

ACTION SHEET

DATE	DETAILS OF THE PROBLEM/CHANGE	WHAT YOU ARE GOING TO DO, OR HAVE ALREADY DONE, ABOUT THE PROBLEM/CHANGE	INITIALS

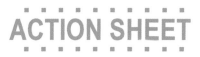 # ACTION SHEET

DATE	DETAILS OF THE PROBLEM/CHANGE	WHAT YOU ARE GOING TO DO, OR HAVE ALREADY DONE, ABOUT THE PROBLEM/CHANGE	INITIALS

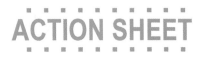

ACTION SHEET

DATE	DETAILS OF THE PROBLEM/CHANGE	WHAT YOU ARE GOING TO DO, OR HAVE ALREADY DONE, ABOUT THE PROBLEM/CHANGE	INITIALS

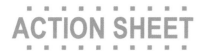

ACTION SHEET

DATE	DETAILS OF THE PROBLEM/CHANGE	WHAT YOU ARE GOING TO DO, OR HAVE ALREADY DONE, ABOUT THE PROBLEM/CHANGE	INITIALS

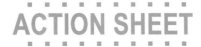

ACTION SHEET

DATE	DETAILS OF THE PROBLEM/CHANGE	WHAT YOU ARE GOING TO DO, OR HAVE ALREADY DONE, ABOUT THE PROBLEM/CHANGE	INITIALS

If you have used all the Action sheets in your pack, photocopy this one before you fill it in, or download new copies from **food.gov.uk/childminders**

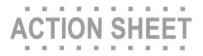

ACTION SHEET

DATE	DETAILS OF THE PROBLEM/CHANGE	WHAT YOU ARE GOING TO DO, OR HAVE ALREADY DONE, ABOUT THE PROBLEM/CHANGE	INITIALS

3-MONTHLY REVIEW

The 3-monthly review is an important part of the records you need to keep about food to comply with the law.

Every three months you should look back at previous months and identify any problems. If you had a serious or persistent problem (the same thing went wrong three times or more), make a note of it below and also write down what you are going to do, or have already done, about it.

There might also have been changes in the way you are working with food e.g:

• Have you changed the ingredients, types of food or recipes you use?

• Are you looking after a new child? Do they have any allergies or need different foods?

• Are you using any different equipment?

If there have been any changes like these, you will need to review your safe methods to make sure they are up to date. Make a note of what has changed below and give details of any changes you need to make to your safe methods.

If you need a new copy of a safe method, you can download one from **food.gov.uk/childminders**. Remember to sign and date the safe method after you have filled it in.

DATE	3-MONTHLY REVIEW COMPLETED	DETAILS OF A SERIOUS OR PERSISTENT PROBLEM OR A CHANGE IN THE WAY YOU ARE WORKING	WHAT YOU ARE GOING TO DO, OR HAVE ALREADY DONE, ABOUT THE PROBLEM OR ANY CHANGES YOU NEED TO MAKE TO YOUR SAFE METHODS
25.06.15	☑	Have a new baby in my care (Richard Brown).	Need to change the 'Babies and children – special advice' safe method to show how I store made-up formula milk provided by the parents.
25.06.15	☑	No problem / changes	No action to take
	☐		
	☐		

3-MONTHLY REVIEW

DATE	3-MONTHLY REVIEW COMPLETED	DETAILS OF A SERIOUS OR PERSISTENT PROBLEM OR A CHANGE IN THE WAY YOU ARE WORKING	WHAT YOU ARE GOING TO DO, OR HAVE ALREADY DONE, ABOUT THE PROBLEM OR ANY CHANGES YOU NEED TO MAKE TO YOUR SAFE METHODS
	☐		
	☐		
	☐		
	☐		
	☐		
	☐		

Printed in Great Britain
by Amazon

46669859R00025